EASY HEALTHCARE:
YOUR HOSPITAL STAY

By

Lori-Ann Rickard

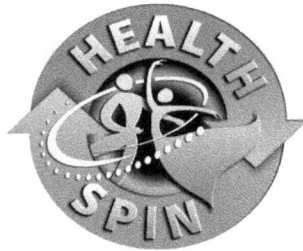

Presented by
Expert Health Press

Visit the Author Website at www.myhealthspin.com

ISBN-10:1940767067
ISBN-13:978-1-940767-06-2

For Asimina, Kristen and Patrick,
for your unwavering support.

TABLE OF CONTENTS

INTRODUCTION

Although we would all like to avoid it, it's likely that most of us will at some point be admitted to the hospital. Sometimes you have the luxury of choice – you're having elective surgery or are being admitted for a test. But in other, more frightening, times you may experience a life-threatening accident or illness and are admitted immediately. Whether you are staying in a hospital for a happy event, such as the birth of a child, or are being admitted due to an emergency or serious illness, you should understand how a hospital works. Knowing what to expect during a hospital stay will make your time there easier.

So, what are the 11 things you need to know about navigating a hospital stay?

1.

CHOOSE YOUR HOSPITAL WISELY

The first thing you should do before you are ever admitted to a hospital is research the hospitals in your area. Most people simply assume that they should go to the one closest to their home. Although this might seem convenient, that hospital may only handle relatively minor problems and may not be equipped to handle a serious emergency or complex illness. You may also find that none of your doctors practice there. So, a little research up front before you or your loved ones ever need to be admitted will save you time, money, and stress in the long run.

Many people assume that every hospital is the same. This is simply not true. There are world-renowned hospitals with extensive funding, prominent staff, and cutting-edge technology; and there are poor hospitals that struggle to meet the needs of the community they serve. There are hospitals affiliated with universities or religious groups. There are hospitals that are for profit and some that are not for profit. All of these distinctions will change your hospital experience.

Also, as they compete for your healthcare dollar, hospitals are focusing more on customer service and the "patient experience." Some present themselves like high-end resorts, with glossy advertisements, impressive lobbies, and waiting rooms with wi-fi and flat screen televisions. But remember, you aren't looking for a great "hotel" to stay at for a few days. You're choosing a hospital that will impact your life. Making the wrong choice can be a decision that could cost you dearly.

CHECK THE HOSPITAL'S REFERENCES

The most important consideration in choosing a hospital is the competency of the doctors and nurses who work there. How good are they at what they do? Often patients who want to control their healthcare experience choose their doctor first, and then follow that doctor to the hospital where he or she practices (we'll discuss more about where a doctor has "credentials" below).

So, consider the credentials of the doctors who may treat you or your loved one. Where were they trained? Are they board certified? A doctor goes to medical school and then does a residency in a specialty. If he or she wants to continue their education, they might do a fellowship in a very specific specialty such as gynecology-oncology or pediatric surgery. Also, a doctor can do his or her training in many locations. Are they trained in the United States? Also, consider how rigorous a doctor's training has been. It's more difficult to get into some medical schools, residencies, and fellowships than others.

If you look at your doctor's educational history, you'll likely get an idea of what type of skills he or she has. For example, if the surgeon who may operate on your baby doesn't have a fellowship in pediatric surgery or similar specialized training, you should ask why.

After a doctor graduates from his or her fellowship, he or she can take a test specific to their specialty, which is called their "boards." A doctor is not required to be "board certified" to practice, but by passing the exam he or she will have a higher level of credentials than someone who has not. This is in part because "board-certified" doctors must periodically retake the exam to keep their certification and prove that they are current with changes in their field. Some hospitals require that all doctors who practice in the hospital be "board certified."

Another factor to consider is the hands-on experience of the doctors at the hospital. For example, if you are having surgery, does the anesthesiologist understand how to care for a patient like you? At a pediatric hospital, a pediatric anesthesiologist handles anesthesia for children every day. However, in a hospital that mostly treats adults, anesthesiologists will only rarely administer anesthesia to a baby. This is important information to know. Unlike most doctors, you cannot pick your anesthesiologist. Your surgeon does. So, it's important that you feel you can trust him or her to know if the anesthesiologist is skilled to handle your care.

WHAT IS THE OVERALL REPUTATION OF THE HOSPITAL?

Every hospital has at least some great healthcare providers working for them; however, you should know what the overall reputation of the hospital is. A good place to start your research is on the Internet, and it will not take long for you to determine what hospitals have great ratings and what hospitals do not. However, as always, beware of believing all the information you see. Look at a variety of reputable sources. Also, don't be misled by the name of the hospital. For example, just because a facility is called "Smith Cancer Treatment Centers," don't assume that it provides better specialty care than a local research hospital.

Also, know that there is no one specific requirement you should be looking for. Instead, consider whether the hospital has the right mix of requirements that are important to you. Examples might include:

- Is it close to home?

- Does your primary doctor practice at that hospital?

- Is there a specialist who you trust there?

- Is the hospital a research hospital?

- Does it have or not have a religious or academic affiliation that is important to you?

- Is it a for-profit or not-for-profit hospital?

For example, if one of your children will be in the hospital for some time, it will be much easier for you to care for your other children at home if the hospital is located nearby. However, this is only one factor, and not always the most important. No matter how close the hospital is, you'll likely be at the hospital most of the time and will need to find family and friends who can help you care for your other children. If the local children's hospital is the best choice for your child's illness, and it is where your child's specialist works, then driving another ten minutes to get there should not be the determining factor.

You should also be aware of what services hospitals in your area offer and which hospitals your doctors practice at. We all know of hospitals that don't provide a full complement of care. For example, the hospital closest to you may be a small, local one that does not have the specialized services you need. Additionally, as mentioned above, most doctors only work at certain hospitals. For example, if your doctor is employed by a hospital system, it's likely the only one where he or she will have credentials. If you do go to a hospital where your doctor is not credentialed, you will be assigned an unknown primary care physician who is.

Additionally, you should understand that your primary care physician or your pediatrician will likely only refer you to specialists who work at the same hospital as he or she does. So, for example, if your child has a heart condition and your pediatrician works at the local community hospital, you will likely have to expand your search beyond his or her recommendations to find specialists at area pediatric or research hospitals.

That being said, your primary care doctor can still be an excellent source of information about local hospitals. If you want your primary care doctor to follow your care while you are in the hospital, you will want to pick a hospital where he or she practices.

SYNCH UP YOUR DOCTORS AND YOUR HOSPITAL

If you choose a hospital where your doctor practices, it can make a stay in the hospital easier. Your recent tests will likely be available, your doctor will know your health history, and staff can more easily coordinate your care. For an individual with a variety of specialists in addition to a primary care physician, having the majority work out of the same hospital system can be especially important.

This is one of the reasons why, as I cared for my aging parents, I insisted that we only select doctors who worked within one hospital system. Because we live in an urban area with several health system choices, I was able to select doctors who worked at a hospital with a good reputation that was also close by our home. However, this also meant that my parents had to, in some cases, switch to new providers.

This was hard for my parents who had seen some of their healthcare providers for years. However, I knew that by making the change while they were healthy, I could ensure better care when they were sick. When their health began to decline there was no question as to what hospital I should take them. And, instead of constantly running to get records from other providers, I knew their doctors could access their health histories without any issues.

Having healthcare providers who know you is especially important as you age. Although it's unfortunate, many seniors enter the hospital with no support system. So, it's easy for a doctor seeing them for the first time to assume that the senior's symptoms are a result of just being old. Many people as they age develop a variety of health problems but are still mentally competent. Until the day he died, my father was a very intelligent, able person. However, at times, if he was having various health issues, he could appear to have a form of dementia or other mentally disabling illness. It was important that he saw the doctors he knew so that when he had a change in his mental capacity the doctors would look further than simply deciding he was old.

TRANSFERRING TO A DIFFERENT HOSPITAL IS RARELY AN OPTION

Once you have been seen in one hospital's emergency room, it's very difficult to be transferred to a different hospital. When an emergency room doctor treats you, he or she is in charge of your care. In almost all circumstances, that doctor will want to admit you to either the hospital you are at or, if you need a higher level of care, to a larger hospital affiliated with their emergency room.

If you believe that you or your loved one is at the wrong hospital, you should immediately start the transfer process. In order to be transferred, you will need a doctor's order, but you should know that doctors are very hesitant to agree to a transfer simply due to a patient's personal preference. In some cases you will be transferred no matter what your preference. Certain types of insurance require that when a patient is admitted to an out-of-network hospital, he or she must be transferred when stable to a facility that is covered by that insurance plan. This may take some time and you may have to pay out-of-pocket for some of the costs. This is why it is simply better to go to the right hospital in the first place.

THE BOTTOM LINE...

- Before you ever need to be admitted, research local hospitals and the doctors who may treat you.

- Consider what the overall reputation of the hospital is.

- Ask your primary care doctor for recommendations.

- Consider a variety of factors when choosing the hospital.

- Know that transferring to a different hospital after you have been admitted is rarely an option.

2.

STARTING IN THE EMERGENCY ROOM (AVOID IT IF YOU CAN)

If you have gone by ambulance to the emergency room or have decided that the emergency room is your only option, you should be prepared for what to expect. For a life-threatening illness or accident, the emergency room is absolutely the best place to be. Most hospitals have the staff and facilities necessary to manage most life-threatening situations in the most effective and efficient manner possible. In a life-threatening emergency, minutes matter. However, if you do not have a life-threatening illness, you should know what to expect and what to bring if you choose to go to the ER.

BRING YOUR HEALTH HISTORY (MEDICAL LIFE LIST)

One of the most important factors in receiving good medical treatment is knowledge of your health history. How a healthcare professional approaches various symptoms is partially based on what he or she knows about the illnesses or conditions you have and the results of recent tests. If the healthcare provider knows nothing about you, he or she will need to start from scratch. Although health information technology is developing, the healthcare industry has not yet evolved to the point where someone can access your health history from any location. This is the primary reason why it's so important for you to keep an updated record that contains all of your important health history, something we call your Medical Life List, including any surgeries, medications, allergies, and procedures. Even if you have that complete list, it's likely that the emergency room doctor will want to repeat various tests or procedures, for which you will be charged.

Also, it's very unlikely that your primary care doctor will come to the emergency room to see you. If you are in a hospital where your primary care doctor is credentialed, he or she will see you once are admitted to the hospital. However, if your primary care doctor does not work at the hospital you have chosen, doctors whom you do not know will see you.

You should know that emergency room doctors are there to treat true emergencies. If your situation is not an emergency, they won't see you until after they've treated more critical patients. These doctors are backed up by a team of specialists who are "on call" to come into the emergency room if needed. So, in the case of a serious accident or life-threatening illness, these specialists will be immediately available. Not so if your condition is not serious. Even if you're feeling terrible with a non-urgent flu virus, it's highly unlikely that a doctor is going to come to the emergency room in the middle of the night or on a weekend to see you. What will happen is that, after a long wait, the emergency room doctor will either send you to your primary care doctor when his or her office opens or provide you with some limited care until that time. Moreover, the bill for this will be generally very expensive, and you'll be expected to pay even if it was only to be sent to your primary care doctor.

THE "WAIT" IN THE ER WILL BE LONG

If you choose to go to the emergency room and you do not have a life-threatening illness, it's likely that you'll wait a very long time to receive care. Because the emergency room is equipped to handle life-threatening illnesses as quickly as possible, the emergency room must triage each patient to determine if he or she needs immediate care. Because there is no way for the emergency room to determine how many patients they'll have at any given time, they must see the sickest patients first. Therefore, even though you aren't feeling well, you may have to wait a very long time to receive the various tests and exams that you need before someone can treat you.

For example, if you're an elderly patient who fell and needs an x-ray, you will not be seen when you first arrive in the emergency room. The emergency room must first attend to those who arrive gravely injured from car accidents, house fires, and shootings. Many of these events occur during the evening hours or on weekends. If you happen to arrive Friday at 8:30 pm and a serious car accident occurred at 8 pm, it's likely that the hospital will be focused on the individuals involved in the car accident for quite some time. It is not unusual to spend more than twenty-four hours in an emergency room waiting for a specific doctor or a test to determine what care to provide. Waiting a long period of time in a cold, sterile emergency room isn't easy when you don't feel well.

HOSPITALS MOVE SLOWLY EVENINGS AND WEEKENDS

Another important piece of information to know is that everything moves slower at a hospital in the evenings and on weekends. There is less staff available, generally, in the emergency room for tests such as x-rays or MRIs. Further, if your illness can wait, the emergency room will likely conduct the tests you need, but send you to see a specialist Monday morning. Often, that specialist will want different tests, and you will be charged for both sets of tests.

CAN YOU HOLD OFF AND SEE YOUR DOCTOR FIRST?

Before you ever step foot into the ER, you should evaluate whether or not you can wait to see your doctor first. For example, my eighty-five-year-old father fell and broke his hip on a Sunday. Although he was in a great deal of pain from what we thought might be a fractured hip, he was otherwise fine. First, we called his primary care doctor to get his advice. As a result, rather than taking a trip to the emergency room and waiting twelve hours for an x-ray that his doctor was unlikely to use, we chose to wait until Monday morning to go to see the orthopedic surgeon. That morning, we went to the office, determined that his hip was fractured, and scheduled him for surgery. For a very independent, proud man, it was much more comfortable for him to be in his house with family on Sunday evening rather than in a cold emergency room where very little care would be provided. This is simply one example of being responsible for your own healthcare needs and making a rational determination regarding what care is necessary and what's truly an emergency.

BEWARE OF OBSERVATION CHARGES

Most people believe that once you enter a hospital you are "admitted" to the hospital. In most cases, this assumption makes sense because you're physically in the hospital when you go to the emergency room. However, you should know that being in the emergency room does not mean you're "admitted" to the hospital. This is very important to understand because your insurance may not cover some of your care if you are not admitted.

Many emergency rooms have a designation called "observation." If you are deemed to be in observation, your insurance will treat you as an outpatient. For many people, especially seniors, this designation can be very expensive. Under Medicare, there is a limit on how much the hospital will be paid for outpatient services. You could be getting the same care after being admitted to the hospital and Medicare would cover the services.

So what is observation? Observation is a status determined by the hospital that means you are too sick to go home but not sick enough to be admitted to the hospital. Observation status requires a doctor's order, and you could be in the emergency room in observation for several days. The hospital may be running several tests in order to determine whether you should go home or be "admitted" to the hospital. Medicare guidelines suggest that "observation" should be limited to twenty-four to forty-eight hours. However, many hospitals hold patients in observation status for several days.

Because Medicare considers observation to be an outpatient service, the senior will have to pay a co-pay and deductible for the doctor's fees. Additionally, he or she will have to pay hospital charges for any routine medications they currently take if they are prescribed while in observation.

Further, it is very important to understand that a Medicare

patient in observation will not have coverage for nursing care or rehabilitation even though a doctor may order it. Such care generally needs to be preceded by a hospital admission. In order to be eligible for nursing care or rehabilitation, the Medicare patient must have spent three consecutive days (midnight to midnight) admitted to the hospital, not including the day of discharge.

Medicare does not require hospitals to inform patients when they are in observation status. The only way to know is to ask. Medicare patients also often believe they've been admitted when in fact they have not. Your doctor may even agree that you need to be admitted, but the decision is ultimately made by the hospital. So, it's important to be proactive, which can be difficult when you aren't feeling well. This is another reason why you must bring someone with you when you go to the hospital to act as your advocate, asking questions and finding out the answers.

Most hospitals have a patient advocate office or ombudsman office. If you aren't getting the answers you need, you should ask to speak with someone who is available to assist patients with getting the answers they need. Remember, waiting to find out your status until you are discharged from the hospital is too late. If you're a Medicare patient there are ways to appeal your bill once it is received; however, it's much more difficult to get the decision changed after the fact.

THE BOTTOM LINE...

- Bring your health history (Medical Life List).

- If your doctors don't practice at the hospital, no one in the ER will likely know you and they will not have access to your medical records.

- If you have an illness or condition that is not life threatening, you will likely wait a long time to be seen.

- Before going to the ER, evaluate if you can first see your doctor at his office.

- Hospitals move slowly in the evening and on weekends.

- Rather than admitting you, hospitals can designate you as staying in "observation," which may be very costly.

3.

ASK TO BE DIRECTLY ADMITTED

Many patients aren't aware that it's possible to be admitted to a hospital without having to go through the emergency room. The hospital must have a direct admit policy and your doctor must provide an order specifically admitting you to a hospital room. Every hospital has its own policy on how to handle directed admissions.

AVOID THE HASSLE AND WAIT OF THE ER

As we have discussed, going to the emergency room can be a long and very frustrating experience. If you know you're going to be admitted to the hospital, going directly to your room is a much better option. However, some hospitals require that you go through the ER first. This is especially true if you are in need of oxygen, IV fluids, or urgent tests.

DISCUSS WITH YOUR DOCTOR

If you're interested in being directly admitted to your hospital room, you should discuss the options with your doctor. In some cases, he or she may be opposed to the idea, and, if so, will not grant the order. Generally, your doctor knows best, but if he or she objects to directed admission, you should ask why. Most likely they are concerned that you won't get the appropriate immediate care you need, so he or she will require you to go through the emergency room.

DIRECT ADMISSIONS HAPPEN ON WEEKDAYS

Most hospitals will only allow direct admissions during certain time periods, usually on a weekday and generally before certain times of day. For example, many hospitals will not allow direct admissions after 4 pm. This is because most hospitals have less staff in the evenings and weekends to handle the paperwork associated with admitting you to the hospital.

THE BOTTOM LINE...

- Being admitted directly avoids the hassle, wait and expense of the ER.

- The hospital you choose must have a direct admissions policy.

- You will need your doctor to write an order.

- Most hospitals only allow direct admissions to occur at certain times of the day and week.

4.

CONSIDER WHAT TYPE OF ROOM YOU WANT

Depending on the reason for your hospitalization, you may be able to choose the type of room you have during your stay. Different rooms have different costs so make sure to inquire about pricing. Also, know what your health insurance provider is willing to cover. For example, most insurance plans will not pay for the entire cost of a private room, so if you make that choice, you will likely pay a portion of the cost yourself.

Also, your circumstances may require you to stay in a specific part of the hospital. You could find out that with your type of illness you can only go to one type of room in one location of the hospital. For example, if you are admitted to the Intensive Care Unit (ICU), you are likely very sick. An ICU requires very specialized equipment in each room and has very specific rules regarding visitors. Therefore, if you are going to the ICU, you will not have much choice.

SEMI-PRIVATE ROOMS

Before being admitted to the hospital, ask what the various choices are regarding rooms. Make sure to ask prior to getting a room assignment. If you find out you were being given a certain room, ask immediately what type of room it is. It is much more difficult to move rooms later.

Every hospital offers different room choices. Normally, there are three types of rooms. In older hospitals, they sometimes still have a "ward-type" room. A "ward" room will often have four patient beds with one or two shared bathrooms. The most common type of room is a "semi-private" room. A "semi-private" room will have two patient beds with one shared bathroom. A curtain usually divides room, offering very little privacy in reality.

In this configuration you likely won't have a choice of who your roommate is, so you should consider how having one will or will not make your stay restful. You could get a great roommate who is quiet and pleasant, or you could be in the bed next to someone who talks incessantly and keeps the television on continuously. Also, while the hospital will certainly not put you in a semi-private room with someone who could get you sicker, remember that with roommates come their visitors and their germs.

PRIVATE ROOM?

There are many benefits to having a private room while staying in the hospital. First, if you plan on having a loved one or friend with you during your hospital stay, it's often easier to have company in a private room. A private room will also provide some type of couch or pull-out chair for your company to sleep on during the evening. Anyone who's been a patient's caregiver knows it can be very exhausting so a place to rest is very important.

Another important consideration regarding a private room is the use of the bathroom. It may be unpleasant to share a bathroom with a stranger when you are not feeling well. This is especially true if you or your roommate need assistance using the bathroom and must call a nurse's aid for help.

WAIT LIST?

If you have a particular preference regarding the type or location of a room and that preference is unavailable, always ask hospital personnel if you can be placed on a wait list. The chances of something opening up can be slim, but patients leave the hospital all the time, and a private room, for example, may become available during your hospital stay. It never hurts to ask.

THE BOTTOM LINE...

- Before you get a room assignment, ask what types of rooms are available.

- Ask what the costs are for the various types of rooms available.

- Consider paying more for a private room if having a roommate would keep you from getting the rest you need.

- If a private room is not currently available, ask if you can move when one becomes available.

5.

PICKING YOUR SPECIALISTS

Whether you arrive at the hospital via the emergency room or direct admission, you need to determine who your specialist will be. If you go to the emergency room, it's likely you'll be assigned a specialist from the hospital. Most hospitals have "trauma call," which means that certain doctors have agreed to be available on a rotating basis for different emergencies. So, if you need immediate attention, the hospital will choose your specialist. If, however, you're having elective surgery or have some time to evaluate and choose your specialist, you should do so.

CONTACT YOUR PRIMARY CARE PHYSICIAN FOR RECOMMENDATIONS

Your primary care physician is a great resource for recommendations regarding a specialist for your specific illness or condition. For instance, if you have broken a hip, you will need an orthopedic surgeon who specializes in hips. If your primary care physician works at the hospital you've been admitted to, a quick call to his office will likely get you the name of a reliable candidate. Otherwise, the hospital will likely assign you to the orthopedic surgeon who happened to have been on call at the time.

CHECK YOUR SPECIALIST'S CREDENTIALS AND REFERENCES

If your primary care physician is unavailable, you may want to do some research on the specialist being recommended to you by the hospital. To begin, most hospitals have a physician directory, which will give you some basic information about the physician.

The Internet will also be a source of information about the physician. However, be careful not to trust all the information on the Internet, as it isn't necessarily credible. Other healthcare providers in the area may be a resource. For example, if you know a nurse or therapist who works at the hospital, they may have very good insight.

It's important to remember that you're not necessarily looking for a physician who has a "winning" personality. You're not selecting a "friend" or "buddy." You're looking for a physician who is very good at what he or she does. Many specialists work long hours under a great deal of pressure. You want someone who will take your problem very seriously and treat it as if it's his or her own.

COMMUNICATION IS KEY

One important skill for all physicians is communication. The physician must be reasonably available and willing to talk to you about any of your concerns. If you have time, it's important to discuss this issue with the physician prior to selecting him or her. Don't expect that your physician will be available twenty-four hours a day, seven days a week, via cell phone. However, you should expect there to be a clear procedure for contacting the physician and getting your questions answered in a timely manner.

Effective communication may sound like a very basic requirement, but it can be one of the most difficult aspects of being a patient. Doctors make their rounds to see their hospitalized patients at very early hours in the morning and are very busy during the day. They often have a variety of surrogates to assist them in seeing their patients. Often, a surrogate such as a nurse practitioner can be of great assistance to the patient in getting basic information about his or her care. However, sometimes the patient actually wants to talk to the physician. You need to make this clear to your nurse and to your doctor's helpers.

THE BOTTOM LINE...

- Check your specialist's credentials.

- Check with friends and family in order to get references.

- Check with your primary care physician for recommendations.

- You are not selecting a "friend" or "buddy," but an excellent physician who can effectively treat your illness or condition.

- Effective communication between the physician and you and your family is key.

6.

MANAGING YOUR STAY

Once you choose your hospital, it's important to consider how you and your loved ones will manage your experience. Never expect the hospital to care for every aspect of your stay while you're there. You or your loved ones must have a plan. By reviewing this section you can be prepared to understand what's happening and know how to follow up with staff on anything that may be confusing or unclear.

Have Someone with You Whenever Possible

Some people believe that when their loved one is in the hospital, staff is with them twenty-four hours a day. Although hospitals provide care around the clock, the nurses and doctors have many patients to care for. Due to cost cutting and various other changes in healthcare, it's becoming more and more difficult for the nurses and doctors to attend to every patient's needs. This is one of the reasons why you should have someone with you at all times, if possible, to act as your advocate and take care of the small things you need. A family member, close friend, or a combination of both can be essential to receiving the care you need. Even if you cannot have somebody with you at all times, it's important to have somebody with you as often as possible, especially when you see the doctor. When you're sick, it's not the best time to attempt to coordinate your care on your own or keep track of the many details associated with your hospital stay.

Beware of Germs

Not surprisingly, hospitals have lots of germs. Although the hospital will do everything possible to prevent you from getting the illnesses of other patients, it's important that you do your part. You should not have any visitors who are sick and let family and friends know to keep small children at home. It's often helpful to keep alcohol wipes with you to sanitize anything that might be brought into the room. Also, your visitors should always wash their hands when they come into the room. Remember you're sick. That means that your immunity is low and your body is trying to fight off the illness. The last thing you want to do when in the hospital is to get sicker due to the people around you.

TAKE NOTES

If possible, you should have someone taking notes about who comes and goes from your hospital room. There are many different healthcare providers who will visit your room and you should know who those individuals are, what their specialties are, and how they think you're doing each day. A hospital day is a very long for a patient. It can be very difficult to remember when people come and go, whether you have gotten the results of the various tests being run, and what the prognosis is for your stay.

A hospital employs many different healthcare providers. Although somebody may walk into your room who appears to be a doctor, he or she may simply be a medical student in training. Hospital training programs dictate that interns and residents come to your room first. An intern is still in medical school, while a resident has graduated from medical school and is being trained in his or her specialty. The interns and residents gather all the data regarding your status and report it to the doctor in charge of your care.

It's important for you to understand who these people are since you'll be more interested in your own doctor's opinion than in their opinions. If you attempt to get the opinion of every intern and resident, you'll rapidly become confused about your care. Your doctor will ultimately decide how to proceed with your care and may not listen to the opinions of the intern or resident. Indeed, it's easy to focus on the opinions of the intern or resident since he or she is likely to take more time with you while your doctor is busy trying to get his or her hospital rounds done each day.

Once your doctor visits, you'll often need to stop him or her to ask your questions. Some attending doctors will actually stand in the doorway of the room to discuss your care. That way, they can see patients quickly. If this happens and you have questions, simply ask them to come into the room. The doctor may say that he or she is busy and will come back later. While you need to be sensitive to the fact that your doctor has many responsibilities, getting answers to your questions is part of caring for you. Since the attending doctor will be billing every day he sees you in the hospital, you are entitled to answers to your questions. You may also want to write down your questions (or have your loved one do so) in advance of seeing the doctor.

THIS IS NOT THE "LOTTO"

I live and work in a large metropolitan area. In the past I had a job that involved interviewing patients who came to the emergency room of a local hospital. When I spoke to them, patients would often say they were "going to the 'lotto'" for a bad cold or other illness. When I finally asked what the "lotto" was, I was told that people saw going to the ER the same as playing the "lotto" because they might be able to bring a lawsuit related to their care and get some money. Although this is certainly not the norm, it's important to remember that the majority of hospital staff take their work very seriously. They are putting in long hours under a great deal of stress, and often their actions can result in life or death. You should understand that they are very concerned about patients who appear to be looking for ways to intentionally bring a malpractice lawsuit for money. Thus, physicians may become concerned if they see you or your family taking notes or pictures to document your care.

Therefore, it's important to use caution when you are taking notes. Knowing that you want to have a good relationship with your doctor, make sure he or she understands the reasons for the note-taking. Simply explaining that the notes help keep the family members who rotate in and out of your room coordinated should help to put your doctor's mind at ease. If you want to take pictures, you should explain why you are taking those pictures before doing so. For example, it may be helpful to refer to a picture of swelling in your feet when you talk to the primary care doctor you might not see for some time. These truthful explanations will help the doctor understand that you're not simply documenting your care so you can later sue him or her.

If for some reason you don't feel comfortable with the doctor and feel compelled to take pictures and notes to document care for a later lawsuit, it's best to change doctors immediately. Trust is one of the most important aspects of the doctor-patient relationship. Also patients need to have realistic expectations. Some individuals believe that healthcare providers have a magic wand and can fix any problem by merely putting a patient in the hospital, but this is rarely the case. If you've smoked for thirty years, are obese, or have never exercised, you'll likely have health conditions that aren't going to be solved by a single visit to the hospital.

ASK QUESTIONS

If you're in the hospital for surgery, you may be visited not only by your surgeon but also by another surgeon from his or her group or practice who will check your status on his or her behalf. Keeping track of names will help you to determine whom you need to talk to if you have a question or concern. A simple way to do this is to merely ask for the doctor's card or ask them to spell their name. You should specifically ask what type of doctor they are. Knowing which group is in charge of decisions about your kidneys versus your heart issues will help you to know who to talk to for what problem.

Knowing when your doctor will be making rounds is important as well. Many doctors do hospital rounds early in the morning. Surgeons often start their operations early in the morning and perform them late into the evening. So, he or she may try to get patient rounds done before surgeries start. If you know the surgeon makes rounds every morning at 6 am, you can plan in advance to have someone with you then and to have your questions organized. If you don't ask them during that visit, it's unlikely that you'll see them again until the next day.

In addition to doctors' visits, you may also be taken from your room throughout the day to get a variety of tests. It's helpful to have a loved one keep track of what tests you're getting and ensure that you get the results of those tests communicated to you. You'd be surprised how many times patients get a variety of tests in the hospital and they have no idea what the tests are for or what their results are. You're paying for each one of these items and you're entitled to know what's being done and what the results are. You and your advocate also need to make sure that all the doctors involved in your care know what tests are being ordered for you.

THE BOTTOM LINE...

- A family member or loved one should be with the patient as much as possible.

- Be careful of unnecessary germs.

- Take notes or have your loved one do so.

- Explain the use of notes or photographs so that the healthcare provider does not think you are documenting for a malpractice lawsuit.

- Don't be afraid to ask questions.

7.

A Day in the Life of a Hospital Patient

Most hospitals have a daily routine. Being aware of the structure of the day often helps with the anxiety of being in a hospital.

NURSES AND AIDES

Each patient room in a hospital generally has both a nurse and an aide assigned to it. Each of these individuals work a certain set time each day. Often, nurses and aides work more than eight hours a day. Your nurse may work three to four twelve-hour periods during the week. Your nurse may also be called to work in a different part of the hospital during their shift. Therefore, you will not have the same nurse or aide each day. However, it's important for you to know who your nurse or aid is at any given time, since he or she can often answer a question or assist you with something that you need.

SHIFT CHANGE

Nurses work a certain amount of hours, known as a shift. Depending on which area of the hospital you are in and the various employees needed throughout the hospital, a nurse will only care for you over a certain period of time. In most hospitals, when a shift starts, the nurse will write his or her name on a board in your room so you can remember who they are for the time they are there. When the nurse goes off shift, they will give a "report" to the next nurse. During the "report," it will be very difficult for you to get much care unless you have an emergency. Therefore, you should make any requests you have prior to the shift change, and then repeat those requests to the new nurse when you first see him or her.

TESTS AND PROCEDURES

You may occasionally be taken from your room to get a test, have a procedure done, or have surgery. Some tests can be performed in your room. For example, an x-ray technician may bring the x-ray machine to your room to take a chest x-ray. Always ask what tests are being performed and why. As with all things regarding your hospital stay, you and your loved ones should take an active part in your care. You know yourself better than anyone else, and if you have questions or feel that a test is inappropriate, you should speak up. A hospital treats hundreds of patients on any given day, and you want to make sure whenever possible that the tests you are getting are necessary and ordered by your physician. Mistakes can happen anywhere and being alert helps to avoid any mix-ups.

HOW DO I EAT?

Meals in a hospital are often an important part of the day. For a patient, the days are very long, and meals offer a way to break up the day and have something to look forward to. Each hospital has a different way of managing patient meals. Old-fashioned hospitals simply deliver a pre-determined meal to your room. In most updated hospitals, you will have a menu to choose from and an ability to order your meals ahead of time.

Also remember that you may have some restrictions based on your illness as to what types of food you can eat. For instance, you may have a low sodium diet or a heart-healthy diet. The kitchen should know what your restrictions are, but, if for some reason, you call the kitchen and they allow you to order something that you aren't supposed to eat, make sure you inform them of your restrictions. Those restrictions are placed on you to help you get better.

If you're very sick, it's nice to have your family member order your meals for the day ahead of time. They can call the kitchen and order those items that you would like from the menu. You should not expect these meals to be "restaurant" grade quality; however, many hospitals have very good food.

If someone is staying with you in the room, you should be sensitive to the fact that your visitor may not be able to eat with you in the room. If you're in the ICU, there will be a limit on how many visitors you can have and it's unlikely that there can food in the room other than yours. This is for the health and safety of all patients and you should respect the hospital's rules. After all, you aren't there to visit with your friends but rather get well and go home.

RESTING IN THE HOSPITAL IS DIFFICULT

When you are sick, you need rest. But hospitals are often the least restful place to be. First, a hospital floor is not quiet. There are many sick people and much work to do. You may hear doctors and nurses attending to other patients, or hospital staff talking amongst themselves. Visitors come and go, televisions are played. Alarms go off, monitoring machines ping. In order to avoid some of the sounds and get some rest, you can request to shut your door. The nurse may or may not let you do so since he or she is responsible for watching you during your hospital stay. If you are very sick and unable to ring your bell for help, it's unlikely you'll be allowed you to shut your door.

Additionally, the hospital staff starts very early in the morning gathering the information they need for the day. This means that you are often woken up very early in the morning for blood work or other tests that the doctors may need during the day to provide care. If your surgery is scheduled very early in the morning, the hospital staff will come get you much earlier than when your surgery is scheduled in order to prepare you. All of these routines are necessary to provide your care; however, it's often difficult to understand why the hospital personnel are waking you up if you are not prepared for the process. Again, asking questions about what to expect will often help you to understand your care.

ALMOST NOTHING OCCURS IN THE HOSPITAL ON THE WEEKEND

One of the more surprising aspects to a hospital stay is that almost nothing occurs on the weekend. Obviously, the ER is running and emergency surgeries are being done. However, if you need routine care such as physical therapy, occupational therapy, or other types of services, they are rarely offered on the weekend. Thus, the weekend can be very long for a patient. This is one of the reasons why if you have the luxury of planning your hospital stay, it's better to come in early in the week and not on a Friday.

THE BOTTOM LINE...

- You will likely have a nurse and an aide assigned to you.

- Ask for anything you need prior to the nursing staff changing shifts.

- Be sure to ask questions if you are taken from your room for other healthcare procedures.

- Have your loved one order meals for you, but don't expect restaurant-quality meals.

- Since resting in the hospital is often difficult, ask if you can shut your room door to minimize noise.

- Almost nothing occurs in the hospital on the weekend, so, if you can, be admitted early in the week.

8.

IMPORTANT PATIENT REMINDERS

Being in the hospital is rarely fun, and it's difficult to go from being independent to relying on others for your basic care. It's important, however, to remember that the hospital has a variety of rules for good reason. The hospital and its employees are trying to keep you safe, get you better, and discharge you from the hospital. Following hospital rules is very important no matter how silly they may seem.

Do As You Are Told

If you are told that you need assistance to sit up, get out of bed, or go the bathroom, abide by those rules. A patient may come into the hospital for a fairly minor problem, but if he or she does not listen to staff, they may end up with a serious injury as a result. For example, you may have come into the hospital because you are dehydrated and as a result disoriented, but if you get up without assistance you may fall and break a bone. Hospital personnel are very cautious because they want to make sure you are not injured further during your stay. Even if you believe you can go to the bathroom on your own, if you were told to ring the buzzer and wait for help, you should do so.

If you are required to stay in bed for a certain period of time during your hospital stay, do so. You'll be very surprised how quickly you become weaker than you normally are. This is another reason why the hospital staff will ask you to ring the buzzer before you get out of bed or use the bathroom.

Following directions is also important when it comes to your diet. The doctors may have put you on a restricted diet while you are in the hospital for variety of reasons. You should only eat those items that the doctor allows. You are in the hospital to get better, and you could make yourself sicker by eating food you've asked your visitors to bring because you're unhappy with hospital food.

Further, you may be asked not to eat at all prior to coming into the hospital if you're having a test or surgery. These rules are very important to your safety and you should follow them exactly as they are given to you (for example, you could vomit while under anesthesia and inhale that vomit into your lungs, causing a serious infection). You do not want to further complicate your illness by violating the rules. If for some reason you forgot to stop eating at midnight as you were instructed, make sure you are honest with the hospital staff upon your arrival. Even if your surgery or procedure must now be postponed, that is better then risking your health.

LIMIT VISITORS

While I strongly encourage everyone to have a family member or friend with them as much as possible during their hospital stay, it's also important to have some limit on your visitors. Remember this is not a vacation or a holiday, and while it's often helpful to have some visitors to brighten the patient's day, too many visitors can be too tiring. You're trying to get better or recuperate from surgery. You need rest and quiet. This is also not the time to bring very small children to the hospital unless you specifically get permission from your doctor. There are very sick people in the hospital and you do not want a child to be exposed to potential infections, nor do you want to be exposed to a child's germs. If you are feeling well enough, a nice compromise may be to go to a lounge in the hospital to have a short visit with your children or grandchildren.

BE FRIENDLY AND COOPERATIVE WHENEVER POSSIBLE

Healthcare providers have a very difficult job. They have many demands on them and rarely have enough time with each of their patients. Generally, their days are very long and filled with stressful problems. You may have a friendly nurse one day and an unpleasant nurse the next. Your doctor may be lovely or may be a person who cannot communicate with a cockroach. No matter whether your healthcare provider is pleasant or not, it's very important for you to be friendly and cooperative. You know the saying: "you get more bees with honey." This is true in every part of the healthcare system.

If you're pleasant and can occasionally overlook a healthcare provider who's having a bad day, you will reap the rewards of receiving better care. No one wants to take care of a patient who's always unpleasant. Remember, you aren't in a hotel where the staff is hired to meet your every need. Every healthcare provider has many patients with different needs and you're just one of them. Try as best you can to do those things for yourself when you are allowed to do so. If your television isn't working, it's not a healthcare crisis. On the other hand, if you feel as though your doctor is constantly unpleasant and unwilling to communicate with you, it may be time to look for a new doctor.

THE BOTTOM LINE...

- Follow hospital rules regarding moving around your room. Don't get up without assistance and stay in bed if told to do so.

- Follow hospital rules regarding food and drink, especially when it comes to surgeries.

- Limit visitors and keep small children at home.

- Be friendly and cooperative with hospital staff whenever possible.

9.

BE PREPARED

It's important that you have the appropriate legal documents completed prior to being admitted to the hospital. This should include a will or a trust. Many people don't want to discuss this because they're uncomfortable talking about being permanently incapacitated or dying. However, no matter how simple the reason may be for you to be admitted to the hospital, it's important to have made your wishes known to your family and loved ones should your care take an unexpected turn. This is especially true as you grow older and the chance for complications rises.

ADVANCED DIRECTIVES

In addition to a will or trust, it's important that you have advance directives, which detail your wishes if you were to become incapacitated. Each state has different rules regarding advanced directives. However, basically, an advanced directive is a written document in which you specify what medical care you want in the future and who you want to make decisions for you should you be unable to make the decisions yourself.

DURABLE POWER OF ATTORNEY FOR HEALTHCARE

A durable power of attorney for healthcare or patient advocate designation, generally, is a document in which you designate a person to make medical decisions for you. This document is often included in your will or trust. The patient advocate will only be able to make decisions for you in the event that you are unable to make them for yourself. Your patient advocate will not be able to take care of other issues that relate to property or finances unless you also designate them to do so in your will or trust. You can also give your patient advocate the power to donate your organs or your entire body upon your death.

LIVING WILL

A living will is a written document in which you inform doctors and family members what type of medical care you wish to receive should you become terminally ill or permanently unconscious. A living will only takes effect once a doctor determines that you are terminally ill and unable to communicate what your wishes are for your medical care.

DO NOT RESUSCITATE

Prior to a procedure, you or your patient advocate may be asked what your wishes are with regard to resuscitation. It may seem silly to you to be discussing such serious issues if you are only going into the hospital for a minor problem. However, it's essential that the hospital knows what your wishes are and has the appropriate documentation just in case. The last thing you want is for a serious problem to occur and your family and the hospital not know exactly what you want done.

Some individuals want all available treatment if they become unconscious. They are willing to be placed on a ventilator or fed through a tube as long as they can stay alive. On the other hand, other individuals want only basic care given, as they do not want to be kept alive by machines. This is an important discussion to have prior to any hospitalization. Upon your admission to the hospital, staff members will ask these questions and document the answers in your medical record. If you have already made these decisions and written them down, it's easy to just give that document to the hospital.

THE BOTTOM LINE...

- You need to be prepared for a life-threatening issue prior to any hospital stay, no matter how simple the original reason for your stay is.

- You should finalize all your advanced directives.

- You should have a durable power of attorney for healthcare.

- You should have a will or trust.

- You should decide whether you want to be resuscitated if necessary.

10.

HAVE A PLAN FOR DISCHARGE

Congratulations! You've survived your hospital stay and the staff is talking about discharging you. It's important that you have a plan for leaving the hospital. If you've gone to the hospital for a minor procedure and will be able to care for yourself upon discharge, there is not much you need to do. Simply find out when you will be discharged and arrange to have someone pick you up. Most people, however, are unable to completely care for themselves once they are discharged from the hospital. Therefore, it's important to have a plan.

TALK TO THE DISCHARGE PLANNER AT THE HOSPITAL

Most, if not all, hospitals have discharge planners who meet with each patient prior to being released from the hospital. The discharge planner may see you at the beginning of your hospital stay to make certain that a plan is in place for when you are discharged. Many people, historically, are readmitted after their hospital stay because they were unable to care for themselves once they left the hospital. Because of new regulations and insurance payment rules, hospitals are making more of an effort to avoid your readmission to the hospital for the same problem.

Also, be aware that the hospital will only want you to stay there for the minimum length of time necessary. When you are admitted, ask your doctors how long he or she expects you to be in the hospital. This will help you plan for your needs after discharge. With so many patients to treat, the hospital cannot let you stay longer while you make a decision on where to go after discharge.

If you are going home, talk to the discharge planner about the possibility of having a visiting nurse or other important health service providers come to your home for some period of time after you are discharged. A home care nurse may visit you several times a week, depending on your condition, to check your health status and provide some limited care. For example, if you have a bandage from your surgery, the home care nurse may be able to change the bandage and make sure that you are healing properly. Additionally, a physical therapist may be able to come to your home to provide some physical therapy if you are unable to drive to their facility.

REHABILITATION FACILITY

Many individuals leave the hospital not for home but for another facility. For example, you may need cardiac rehabilitation after a heart attack so it may be beneficial to go into a specialized rehabilitation facility that can provide such care and closely monitor your progress prior to you returning home. If the discharge planner discusses the possibility of going to a rehabilitation facility, you should ask for a list of possible facilities and have your family or loved one visit the various options while you are in the hospital so you can make an informed decision when the time comes.

NURSING HOME OR ASSISTED LIVING FACILITY

Some individuals may be unable to return to independent living after a hospital stay. If not discussed or expected beforehand, this can be an extremely difficult proposition. Obviously, an illness can arise very suddenly and decisions must sometimes be made during the hospital stay. If the discharge planner and the doctor do not believe that you can return to your home after the hospital stay, you should consider a possible short-term stay in a nursing home or assisted living facility. By arranging for a temporary stay, you and your loved ones can take the time to monitor your condition and make a more informed decision when the pressure to leave the hospital is no longer present. Hopefully, this will be a merely temporary move until you are feeling better and can return to your home. Again, it is important to have your family or friends tour the possible locations in order to make a good decision about where you will go.

A RELATIVE OR FRIEND'S HOME

Another possibility is to stay with a relative or friend upon discharge, or have him or her stay with you in your home. If you know someone who would be able to assist you while you recuperate, this is often the most cost-effective option. Additionally, it may make you feel more comfortable to be with a person you know.

THE BOTTOM LINE...

- Make sure you have a plan for where to go when you are discharged.

- Talk to the discharge planner about options.

- If you return to your home, consider hiring services such as home care nursing and rehabilitation.

- If you must be released to a rehabilitation facility, have loved ones visit and evaluate potential locations on your behalf (or tour them in advance if you know what the expected outcome of your hospital stay will be).

- If the hospital recommends that you go into an assisted living or nursing facility, consider a temporary stay at one first before making a permanent move.

- Determine if you might be able to recuperate in a relative's home or have a loved one stay with you in your home.

11.

WHAT TO DO WITH
THE HOSPITAL BILL

Now you're finally home. In the mail, you receive an enormous hospital bill. What should you do? First, you should be aware that hospital charges very greatly depending on where you are located and what hospital you went to. The first thing you should do is review the bill to determine whether you received all of the services that you were billed for. You would be surprised at how many charges are on a hospital bill that may not relate to your care. Therefore, it's important that you review all of the charges. There may be items on the bill that are appropriate, but you do not understand, so you should call the hospital with any questions you have. If you have insurance, you can also contact your insurance company to clarify any issues regarding your coverage.

Remember these charges matter to you, not just to your insurance company. Many of the charges may not be covered by your health plan, so they will impact your deductible. If you're charged for items that should have been billed to someone else, make sure the charges are taken off your bill. Depending on the type of insurance you have, those charges could make your premium go up in the coming years. Hospitals are notoriously bad at explaining bills to patients and getting the charges right before the bill goes out. Take the time to look at the bill and make a call if you see something that is in error.

You Can Negotiate Your Bill

It's also important to understand that hospitals, for the most part, will negotiate their bills. After completely understanding the bill and determining how much you owe, you should discuss with the hospital a plan for payment. Hospitals will often offer you a payment plan. The hospital may also offer to reduce the bill if you can pay for the services all at one time. Many hospitals also have financial assistance programs.

You should not expect that negotiating your hospital bill will be easy. Hospital bills are historically very difficult to read and understand. It will take a great deal of time and some detective work.

ORGANIZE YOUR BILLS

You will get many bills from many different healthcare providers. In addition to your hospital bill, you will likely get bills from individual doctors you saw in the hospital. Also, you may get bills from doctors you don't remember ever seeing; however, they read your x-rays or reviewed other tests while you were in the hospital. You may want to prepare a spreadsheet to organize everything.

Review each bill carefully to determine if you received the service and whether there are any duplicative charges. In cases where your stay in the hospital was long and complex, you may want to consider hiring someone to assist you in this process as the bills can become very confusing. Since the bill can be very large, hiring an expert may be worth it.

CONTACT YOUR HEALTHCARE PROVIDERS

You have every right to understand what charges are on your hospital bill. It's sometimes beneficial to ask to speak with someone in person about the bills. If you believe that a bill has an improper charge, you should bring it to the healthcare provider's attention. If they refuse to address the problem, you can contact your insurance company, Medicare, or Medicaid.

If you believe that the charges are correct but seem to be excessive, you can ask that the hospital charge you only the portion of the fee that your insurance company has agreed to pay the hospital. For example, Blue Cross Blue Shield may have negotiated with the hospital to only pay 80 percent of the hospital's normal charges. If you have a variety of out-of-pocket costs, you can ask that the hospital only charge you 80 percent of those out-of-pocket costs. The hospital may be willing to negotiate the fee.

REPORT FRAUD

If you review your bills and determine that the charges do not reflect the services you received, you should ask that the hospital remove those charges from your bill. If they refuse, every insurance company, including Medicare and Medicaid, have a hotline to report health care providers who are charging fees that are not appropriate.

THE BOTTOM LINE...

- If you ask, most hospitals will negotiate their bills.

- Ask if the hospital will offer a payment plan (most do).

- Many hospitals will offer financial assistance.

- Get organized. After a hospital stay you will receive a variety of bills from the hospital, providers you know, and providers you never met.

- Contact your healthcare providers to clarify any charges.

- If you see suspect charges and you cannot get a reasonable answer from the hospital or the healthcare provider, report them to your insurance company, Medicare, or Medicaid.

CONCLUSION

Very few people get through life without a hospital stay, and today hospitals are becoming more confusing, complex, and business-like than ever before. Therefore, it's important for a patient to know what to expect before going into the hospital. Having a plan and taking charge of your healthcare while you're a patient will help you better navigate the hospital and get better sooner.

TERMS TO KNOW

Advanced directive: A legal document signed by you that clearly outlines your wishes for life-saving measures and healthcare options that may prolong your life.

Assisted living facility: Residential facility that assists seniors with aspects of daily living while focusing on providing as much independence as possible.

Board certified: Status granted to a medical professional who has proven, through periodic testing by a recognized authority, that she or he has mastery over his or her discipline. Many hospitals require that their doctors be "board certified."

Co-pay: Flat fee an individual pays as an "out of pocket" expense when he or she visits the doctor.

Credentialed: Term referring to a physician's ability to practice medicine at a given hospital. Administrators will regularly review a physician's training, practice history, and certifications among other factors to determine if he or she may practice at their hospital.

Deductible: The amount an individual must spend before a health insurance plan will make payments for his or her healthcare. Some services, for example preventative care, are exempt from the deductible.

Directed admission: Process by which a patient is admitted directly to the hospital rather than through the emergency room.

Durable power of attorney for healthcare: Document in which you designate a person to make medical decisions for you. This document is often included in your will or trust.

Intensive Care Unit: Specialized area of a hospital in which critically ill patients receive comprehensive and concentrated care.

Intern: Physician in training who has not yet graduated from medical school.

Living Will: A document in which you inform doctors and family members what type of medical care you wish to receive should you become terminally ill or permanently unconscious.

Medicaid: A joint federal- and state-funded program that provides healthcare to low-income Americans.

Medicare: Insurance program run by the federal government that provides health coverage to people over the age of sixty five. Medicare also provides coverage for people with certain disabilities as well as those with end stage renal disease.

Nursing home: Facility that provides comprehensive assistance with activities of daily living and continuous medical care.

Observation: Status determined by a hospital that means a patient in the emergency room is too sick to go home, but not sick enough to be admitted to the hospital. Patients under observation may have tests run or be monitored to see if further symptoms develop.

On call: Status in which a physician is ready to respond when needed to care for patients.

Order: A written direction from a physician outlining care for a patient.

Out-of-network: Term used to describe doctors and hospitals that do not accept the contracted rate of an insurance plan.

Out-of-pocket: Costs associated with health insurance plans that are paid by the individual themselves and not the insurance provider.

Patient advocate: The person legally designated by you as the one whom the doctor can communicate with in the event that you cannot participate in your own healthcare decisions. The patient advocate will also know your wishes regarding treatment and end-of-life choices in the case of terminal illness or a serious accident.

Patient advocate office: Department at a hospital that represents patient needs to administrators while assisting patients in resolving individual concerns.

Premium: The monthly price an individual pays to have access to his or her health insurance plan.

Rehabilitation facility: Facility where individuals recovering from serious injury or illness can receive intensive therapy to regain physical strength or rebuild skills such as speaking or walking.

Resident: Physician in training who has graduated from medical school and is learning his or her specialty.

Semi-private room: Type of hospital room with two patient beds and one bathroom.

Trauma call: Status in which a doctor is ready to respond when called to an emergency room.

Triage: Method by which healthcare professionals prioritize which patients should be treated first based upon the relative severity and urgency of the patient's condition.

Ward room: Type of hospital room with commonly four patient beds and one to two bathrooms.

LORI-ANN'S ON YOUR SIDE

"When I need health care advice I can understand and follow, I call Lori-Ann. She knows her stuff!"
M. Diane Vogt, JD

"Lori-Ann is my "go-to" expert on healthcare law. She makes it understandable and easy to follow for our doctors and their patients, too."
Michele Nichols, The Physician Alliance

"Lori-Ann knows the healthcare system inside and out. Whenever we have questions about healthcare, Lori-Ann has the answers."
Mike Gerstenlauer, St. John-Macomb Hospital

"Whenever my family has a health care issue, Lori-Ann is my first call for the best advice."
Donna Curran

"Getting coverage for prescription drugs can be a big problem for patients. Lori-Ann knows the insider secrets to making it easy."
Coreen Buehrer

"Lori-Ann has also lived the difficult issues that families confront on a daily basis as they struggle with the bewildering maze of hospitals, multiple specialists and insurance companies as our family's tireless advocate for our father. No mother grizzly ever fought for her cubs with more passion than Lori-Ann looked out for our dad."
Stephen Rickard, J.D., MPA

ABOUT THE AUTHOR

Lori-Ann Rickard is one of the country's top healthcare lawyers. For over three decades, she has advised leading hospitals, doctors, laboratories, and other healthcare providers. Now she offers her expertise to patients and their families through the Easy Healthcare Series from HealthSpin.

Lori-Ann is also a single mom of two beautiful daughters. One of her daughters was very sick when she was born. Already caring for a toddler and managing a developing career, Lori-Ann used her professional experience to create quick, effective strategies to make the healthcare system work for her as she sought the best treatment possible for her sick baby. Later, Lori-Ann served as the primary caregiver and medical coordinator for her proud, independent parents when they became unable to care for themselves. Through their wellness challenges, her daughter's illness, and in helping friends over the past thirty years, Lori-Ann has used her unique position in the industry to create easy healthcare solutions that work for everyone around her. These solutions will work for you and your family, too.

Lori-Ann Rickard is a healthcare insider who knows what it means to be a patient and a caregiver. The Easy Healthcare Series brings you the benefit of Lori-Ann Rickard's expertise. Let her show you how you can Spin Your Healthcare Your Way.

MORE BY LORI-ANN RICKARD

Visit myhealthspin.com to download your free copy
of *Easy Healthcare: **What You Need First!***

ALSO AVAILABLE FROM HEALTHSPIN:

HEALTH SPIN
Spin Your
Healthcare
Your Way

Easy Healthcare
**BEFORE YOU
GET SICK**

Lori-Ann Rickard, J.D.
Nationally Acclaimed Healthcare Expert

HEALTH SPIN
Spin Your
Healthcare
Your Way

Easy Healthcare
**CHOOSING AN
ASSISTED
LIVING
FACILITY**

Lori-Ann Rickard, J.D.
Nationally Acclaimed Healthcare Expert

HEALTH SPIN
Spin Your
Healthcare
Your Way

Easy Healthcare
**HEALTHCARE
PRIVACY**

Lori-Ann Rickard, J.D.
Nationally Acclaimed Healthcare Expert

HEALTH SPIN
Spin Your
Healthcare
Your Way

Easy Healthcare
OBAMACARE

Lori-Ann Rickard, J.D.
Nationally Acclaimed Healthcare Expert

www.ingramcontent.com/pod-product-compliance
Lightning Source LLC
Chambersburg PA
CBHW050559280326
41933CB00011B/1903